T0297201

COVID-19

Resources for Coping with the Pandemic and Beyond

Dr. Sam Mayhugh &
Dr. Brian Mayhugh

Copyright © 2020 Dr. Sam Mayhugh & Dr. Brian Mayhugh.

All rights reserved. No part of this book may be used or reproduced by any means, graphic, electronic, or mechanical, including photocopying, recording, taping or by any information storage retrieval system without the written permission of the author except in the case of brief quotations embodied in critical articles and reviews.

The information in this book does not provide medical advice. The material is presented for informational purposes only and is not meant to be a substitute for professional medical advice, diagnosis or treatment. Seek the advice of a healthcare provider with questions or concerns regarding a medical condition and/or treatment. Do not delay obtaining medical advice, and do not delay seeking treatment based upon the information contained within this book.

WestBow Press books may be ordered through booksellers or by contacting:

WestBow Press
A Division of Thomas Nelson & Zondervan
1663 Liberty Drive
Bloomington, IN 47403
www.westbowpress.com
1 (866) 928-1240

Because of the dynamic nature of the Internet, any web addresses or links contained in this book may have changed since publication and may no longer be valid. The views expressed in this work are solely those of the author and do not necessarily reflect the views of the publisher, and the publisher hereby disclaims any responsibility for them.

Any people depicted in stock imagery provided by Getty Images are models, and such images are being used for illustrative purposes only. Certain stock imagery © Getty Images.

ISBN: 978-1-9736-9287-4 (sc)
ISBN: 978-1-9736-9288-1 (e)

Library of Congress Control Number: 2020909915

Print information available on the last page.

WestBow Press rev. date: 5/29/2020

WESTBOW
PRESS®
A DIVISION OF THOMAS NELSON
& ZONDERVAN

Dedicated to

the men and women on the front lines working to stop COVID-19

and

to the many souls who have perished in the pandemic

and

Arlene Middleton Mayhugh, loving wife & mother

ACKNOWLEDGEMENTS

This resource book was prepared in response to the effects of the COVID-19 mitigation and containment program on the emotional and mental needs of individuals and families. Several persons contributed to its completion.

Dr. Brian Mayhugh, IBH Chief Clinical Officer, the co-author, contributed clinical information from two large webinars that he developed for over 10,000 companies, dealing with the pandemic impact on employees.

Nora Betancourt, TGA Executive Project Director, conducted research of the personal resources available to persons in quarantine or isolation. She also wrote significant tips and summaries of clinical elements. She offered the dramatic cover design page to the design and production team of West Bow Press.

D. Paul Thomas, friend, actor, essayist, and TGA Creative Director, provided structure, formatting, and editing, while diligently working on TGA's book, soon to be released on Amazon, *"The Odyssey of King David – God's Broken Vessel."*

Dr. Eric Gustafson, IBH Senior Vice President, contributed special material for the depression, resilience, and mindfulness sections.

CONTENTS

PREFACE

There are many motivations for writing a book. I needed none other than the one I received in an email from a woman who worked for me at a behavioral health company I founded thirty-two years ago. She is a psychologist and works in a clinical call center doing telephonic assessment, coaching and referring callers to mental health providers as appropriate. The COVID-19 pandemic has greatly increased the number of calls she receives and the intensity of those calls. In this case, the caller was an employee of a client company that provides employee assistance and mental health services. Desperate, on an early Friday morning, the 25-year-old young man called the 800 number on his health benefit card and spoke to the psychologist.

While my psychologist friend does not drive an ambulance or work in the ER of a hospital, she performed admirably that morning as a "first responder" to a deeply "grieving patient." Her email reads:

"Dr. Sam, I need to share an experience that overwhelmed me last week. Most of you know I work as a mental health clinical case manager. I spend my day talking to people all over the country who need help. Last Friday, my first call of the day was from a 25-year-old man who was sobbing on the phone before I ever said hello. His uncle had died the previous day from Covid-19. He had another uncle who was in ICU and not expected to survive- from Covid-19. His mother and two younger brothers had been told the day his uncle died that they all tested positive. They all lived in the same house, and those still at home were isolating themselves in separate bedrooms.

It was not the loss, impending loss, and feared future loss that had this young man in tears. And it wasn't like that alone was not enough. He was sobbing because he could not grieve "right." He could not be with his uncle who died, nor comfort the one who was about to die. He cannot be with his mother or brothers, they cannot hold each other and cry together and rage against the ravages they have all suffered and may well suffer more of. He sat in a room alone, wondering who would be next, not knowing what to do. He did not know whether he was infected or not.

It was all I could do to not sob with him on the phone. Ok, truth be told, my professional distance crumbled and I did cry. But I hid it from him, and looking back on it, I don't know if that was an awful thing to do. It would have been human to share his tears, sure, but the last thing in the world that needed to happen in the time I spent with him was for him to feel responsible for my tears. I sat there, a stranger on the phone, listening to his grief, his fear, his pain, knowing I could do nothing more than that, and to give him referrals to talk to a local therapist. And pray for him.

When you get restless staying at home and isolating, please remember that the disease is not the only problem here. It's grieving alone, not being able to BE with each other when facing the losses it brings.

I was not sure I was actually going to go back to work today. I did, and I will again tomorrow. Knowing there is little to nothing I can do to help anyone in this situation is hard, and my heart is not as well protected as it used to be. I'm going to be taking a few days off over the Easter weekend to give myself some time and space to grieve and to rebuild those professional boundaries. I've seen some grisly stuff in 24 years as a psychologist. I don't think I have ever felt so wrung out as I do now."

Signed, Psychologist, Case Manager

My friend's email above speaks volumes for the pain and grief that COVID-19 is having on both families and healthcare professionals around the world. May this book help relieve some of that suffering.

Dr. Sam Mayhugh,

April 22, 2020

INTRODUCTION

Before we address the COVID-19 pandemic and its continued impact on us in the United States, it helps to review and understand global pandemics and specifically the 1918-1919 Spanish Flu pandemic. We will especially compare and contrast that pandemic with the 2020 COVID-19 pandemic.

The Antonine Plague of 165AD to 180AD, is estimated to have killed 5 million persons of small pox or measles. It was described by a Greek physician, Galen, who lived in the Roman Empire. It was brought to the Roman Empire by infected soldiers who returned from wars in the Near East.

The Plague of Justinian occurred between 541AD and 542AD. It was caused by bacteria, spread by rats and fleas. The name was given by Procopius of Caesarea who reported that the plague was God's punishment for the Emperor Justinian's evil ways. He also called Justinian a devil. Procopius had studied the plague origins to China and India, by land and sea trade routes to Egypt. There it entered shipping ports. Even though Procopius knew the plague's origins were related to a booming trade and economy, He used "fake news" to blame and embarrass the emperor. Several scholars believe that this plague, wrongly assigned to the emperor, resulted in the destruction of Justinian's plan and attempt to reunite Western and Eastern portions of the Roman Empire. The subsequent period is known as the Dark Ages. From about 500AD until 1400AD. After the collapse of the Roman Empire, also known as the Early Middle Ages, Europe experienced chaos, political and economic destruction, and lost the intellectual/knowledge development that existed prior to the plague and fall of the Roman Empire.

Only 200 years later, the Japanese Smallpox Epidemic hit and killed one million persons. It is believed that smallpox had come to China 200 years earlier, and was then carried to Japan. The epidemic of two years may have killed one-third of the population.

In 1347, the Black Death/Bubonic plague raged on for 4 years. It was a bacteria spread by rats and fleas to humans. It is estimated to have killed 200 million persons, or between 30% and 50% of Europe's population. It took more than 200 years for recovery of the population on the European continent. During this period, efforts were made to protect coastal cities from the epidemics by refusing entry of ships at Venice, and requiring the ships to be anchored for 40 days. Such was the first use of the Italian word "quaranta giorni", or 40 days of quarantine.

In 1520, the smallpox virus was introduced to the Mexican population when Cortes' army fought an army from Cuba, sent to verify that the Spanish plans were on track. The virus killed possibly 56 million of the native population of Mexico and is thought to have allowed Cortes to defeat the Aztec empire, at what is now Mexico City. Following this, a smallpox vaccine was developed.

Between 1600 and the 1800's, a series of plagues hit European cities. Bacteria, borne by rats and fleas killed 3 million, Cholera bacteria killed 1 million, Bacteria borne by rats and fleas killed another 12 million, Yellow Fever, a virus borne by mosquitos, killed 100-150 thousand persons.

1889 to 1890 saw the Russian Flu kill 1 million persons. It is believed to be the H2N2 virus of bird origin.

1918 to 1919 experienced the Spanish Flu, identified as the H1N1 virus, borne by pigs. 40 to 50 million persons died globally. The first awareness was of the virus activity in Spain, and it quickly became named the Spanish Flu. It spread to countries around the world and appeared to be dying out during the first year. But, two more waves of this virus hit and approximately 50 million persons died, of which 675,000 were Americans. It affected 25 percent of the world's population. The case mortality rate was 2.5 percent. Many elements are common with those of the 2019 COVID-19 pandemic. Hospitals added beds in hallways and porches. Temporary hospitals were set up, mortuary services and caskets were insufficiently available. Variance from the COVID-19 pandemic is that approximately 50 percent of the deaths in the second and third waves occurred in 20 to 40-year-olds, and respiratory severity began, often within 2 days of the original symptoms. Jeremy Eichler writes in the May 6, 2020 Boston Globe, about the paucity of works of art, including literature, that are available to remind us later, of the nature and impact of this specific national catastrophe. The events and recording of the overlapping World War I, took top billing and carried forward much memorable material. Eichler points to a particular art piece by Edvard Munch, "*Self-Portrait With the Spanish Flu.*" She describes the self-portrait as "projecting a sense of isolated suffering, an aura of profound loneliness."

With the thousands of persons dying alone in COVID-19, we should determine if memories are sufficiently recorded to convey the pain and suffering of the dying, the anguish of the family members not allowed to comfort, the traumas of the healthcare and government workers, and last but not least the tremendous efforts of many to help and support those affected by both the disease and the impact of the mitigation and prevention actions. Not producing, or losing the elements that remind us of the current pandemic, would be a serious disservice to both current and future generations.

In 1957 - 1958, the Asian Flu, an H2N2 virus, struck and killed over one million persons, including 100,000 in the United States. It originated in China and lasted through 1958.

From 1981 to the present, HIV/AIDS continues. It is a virus with Chimpanzee origin. To date, it has killed 25-35 million persons. It is a human immunodeficiency virus that weakens a person's immune system by destroying important cells that fight disease and infection. To date, there is no effective cure for HIV. But with proper medical care, HIV can be controlled with multiple medications and close medical management.

2002 - 2003 brought SARS, a Coronavirus with origin in bats and civets. It is highly contagious and at times, fatal, as a respiratory disease. It was first seen in China in November 2002. It is a strain of corona virus that causes the common cold. It is believed that the virus mutated in animals and crossed to humans. An outbreak in Hong Kong and slow reporting by China allowed a rapid growth to many other countries, also a criticism of the COVID-19 beginning. Global efforts to contain SARS were successful and it has not been seen since 2004.

2009 - 2010 the Swine Flu hit. It was the H1N1 virus named because it is present in pigs. It was the second pandemic involving H1N1 influenza virus. As a different version, it was responsible for the 1918-1920 Spanish Flu pandemic. It killed 200,000 persons globally. H1N1pdm09 virus was very different from H1N1 version viruses that were present at the time of the pandemic. Older people had developed antibodies against the older H1N1 version and resisted the disease, where young people had not been exposed and therefore had no existing immunity to the new (H1N1) pdm09 virus. Vaccination with the seasonal flu vaccines did not provide cross-protection against (H1N1) pdm09 virus infection. A vaccine was developed after cases in the United States had peaked. It was estimated that there were over 60 million cases, almost 300,000 hospitalizations, and 12,000 deaths in the United States.

2014 - 2016 the Ebola virus originated in wild animals. It infected almost 30,000 and killed 11,000 persons. This particular Ebola outbreak in West Africa was caused by the Zaire strain of the Ebola virus.

2015 to present, MERS, a Coronavirus, originated in bats and camels. It killed 850 persons. Middle East respiratory syndrome MERS-COV is a viral respiratory disease caused by a novel coronavirus. It was first identified in Saudi Arabia in 2012. Typical MERS symptoms include fever, cough and shortness of breath. Pneumonia is common, but not always present, very much like the symptoms of COVID-19. Approximately 35% of reported patients with MERS-COV infection have died. Much of the infections have occurred in human to human contacts in health care facilities but some evidence suggests that dromedary camels are an animal source of MERS-COV infection in humans.

2019 to present, COVID-19 continues. It is a Coronavirus, with possible origin in bats, and generally believed to have originated from China. As of May 7, 2020, 1.23 million cases were counted in the U.S. and over 70,000 persons died.

The takeaways from an historical review of pandemics are:

- Numbers and proportion of populations have declined over time. Rarely, have pandemics extended beyond a few years.
- Earlier, unhealthy living conditions, rats, fleas, birds, and other animals allowed and supported the spread of infections in the population.
- Developing world trade and travel delivered human to human infections from regions to global status.
- Urbanization concentrated people, making infections expand more quickly and proportionally.

- Knowledge of the geography and transmission of infections allowed attempts at containment, including the 40-day quarantine of ships at the port of Venice.
- Currently, the quarantine of individuals and families is used to mitigate or contain the pandemic.
- Evidence of antibodies to one pathogen may provide protection for a similar, but mutated pathogen.
- Effective vaccines can significantly reduce the impact on and deaths of many in the population.

Considering the 2019 COVID-19 Pandemic

Tragically, governments, the health-care industry, and individuals were ill-prepared when COVID-19 sneaked its way onto the world stage. Even those entities that were modestly prepared didn't anticipate the extent nor the intensity of the disease. While early symptoms can range from very mild to severe—a low grade fever, cough, and shortness of breath—the virus frequently leads to an acute respiratory syndrome which leaves its victim gasping for breath and life.

To our best knowledge, the outbreak of the disease began in China in the latter part of 2019. Within months, it had spread to numerous countries and was eventually identified by the World Health Organization as a global pandemic on March 11, 2020. It appears to be shared from person to person when there is close contact or proximity. It is spread by respiratory droplets when someone infected with the virus coughs or sneezes. The droplets remain potent to infect various surfaces for differing times, and place persons at risk of getting the disease when they've come in contact with these contaminated surfaces.

Federal, State, and local governments in the United States have used health recommendations to implement strict regulations in order to mitigate, slow down, and contain the rapid increase of infected persons, and to be able to better treat the alarming number of patients. These efforts have included social distancing, self-quarantine, isolation, and restrictions on travel, business, and social activities. Near total lockdown and shelter-in-place requirements have been mandated across most of the country. Much of the population has been restricted to remaining in homes or locations where persons can be physically separated and in small groups. Churches, social events, and non-essential businesses have been closed. With so many workplaces shut down, millions of employees have been left without financial support, and frequently without health benefits.

This financial uncertainty, social and physical separation, accompanied by the extreme difficulty in obtaining our most basic needs for sustenance, has impacted all of us. Much of our daily routines have changed dramatically. Life as we have known it, will never quite be the same. And regardless of how long these new life situations and patterns continue, it is more important than ever that we have access to the information and resources necessary for our emotional, mental, physical and spiritual health, enabling us to maximize our positive behavioral functioning during these stressful times.

It is our hope that this book will provide you with some information and resources you will need, as we collectively navigate this new, COVID-19 world. Much of the approaches, information, and recommendations contained herein are based on the underlying framework and paradigm of Cognitive Behavior Therapy (CBT). We can use Cognitive Behavior Therapy as a tool to regain control over our changing life, and in the process, change our feelings and thinking, reduce fears, manage stress-related anxiety and depression, and find new ways to cope with the challenges of this new life.

CHAPTER 1

USING CBT TO RESPOND TO LIFE-CHANGES

Dr. Allen R. Miller is a psychologist and the CBT Program Director at the Beck Institute for Cognitive Behavior Therapy. His article in The Beck Institute, *In the News,* takes us from the grief of losing life as we know it to considerations for applying techniques of CBT in some of our responses to the effects of COVID-19:

"The absence of consistent and reliable information about the coronavirus seems to be increasing people's anxiety. They often think, "I don't know what to do"; "Am I doing the right thing"; and "What else should I be doing?" No wonder they feel confused and overwhelmed. Cognitive Behavior Therapy (CBT) is uniquely suited to help people gain control of their lives and feel better. Public health officials have given us directions to maintain physical distance from others, wash our hands for 20 seconds, and disinfect our surroundings. While many people are following those directions, some are not. Following these directives doesn't necessarily alleviate people's fears about what comes next, though. Indeed, there is a lot of uncertainty. We don't know the path of the virus nor its longevity. The destruction that has already been done by the virus doesn't seem to be the full measure of its toll. We have seen people react to the pandemic by trying to gain control of their lives and surroundings. It is the effort to gain excessive control that leads to constant checking and sometimes hoarding of crucial medical supplies.

Paradoxically, the more we try to control everything in our environments, the less control we feel. The infinite number of possible actions is greater than we can calculate, let alone act upon. We need to do what we reasonably can to manage ourselves and our surroundings and ultimately, we need to get comfortable with the idea that we don't have control.

What is the cost of the relentless pursuit of control? Observable behaviors like bulk purchasing and excessive cleaning are the tip of the iceberg. Underlying these behaviors are a range of negative thoughts and painful emotions. CBT tells us that excessive attempts to control are associated with thoughts such as "I am vulnerable," and assumptions that "If I don't over-prepare, then I will fall victim." When we think this way, we feel fear and irritability. When thoughts, emotions and behaviors are aligned in this way, a repetitive cycle begins based on the belief that "There is danger and whatever I do is inadequate." This is the underlying explanation for why trying to gain control only leads individuals to feel less in control.

How do you give up control and how does giving up control help you to feel better? CBT uses a scientific approach to answer these questions. First, question yourself about what sounds reasonable and is founded in scientific evidence. For instance, "Does it make sense and is there evidence to support the effectiveness of recommendations such as social distancing, hand washing, and keeping your hands away from your face?" Alternatively, "Does it make sense and is there evidence to suggest that repeatedly scrubbing your hands for more than 20 seconds will reduce the likelihood of contracting the virus?" Most people conclude that the first question is answered affirmatively and that the second question is not. Listening to public health officials and saying, "I have done everything that is reasonably possible" is a step that illustrates that one is shifting the focus from listening to fear-related thoughts such as "I am in danger," to more realistic thoughts such as "I have followed the recommendations of the scientists who know more about the virus than I do."

The next step can be a difficult one. Unfortunately, doing everything that we possibly can do does not give us absolute control over the virus, or even our immediate surroundings. Even on a good day, we as individuals don't control the world. Whether it's good things that happen to us on a daily basis or a global pandemic, we don't sit in the driver's seat. In spite of the actions we take, we don't control much about our surroundings. This step is accepting at a deep level that we don't have control. In situations when we don't get what we want, or worse, that we get what we don't want, we may feel hurt and angry.

If we give up control, where does that leave us? Well, most of us are left at home isolated from people we know and deprived of activities we like. This is a perfect time to reflect on things we truly value and what is important to us. This is a very individual matter. People may value being productive, providing for their families, spirituality, relationships, activities, the arts, sports, or something else. Which of these that we as individuals value is not the important thing, although we may reassess what we think is important at a time like this.

When we have identified what we value and what is important to us, we are uniquely empowered to pursue those things. CBT tells us that acting according to our values will help us feel better and improve our self-efficacy. We have empowered ourselves to act on those things we have determined are most important to us. By doing so, we give ourselves control. Control— the thing we have wanted all along— is now ours. As we move along this path, it is essential that we keep in mind what we value. What we do and how we do it will be meaningful and have purpose for us when we remind ourselves that we are pursuing our own aspirations.

We can use CBT to reduce our fears, conquer overwhelmed feelings, change our thinking and act in meaningful ways." Allen R. Miller, Ph.D., *Using CBT to Respond to COVID-19,* ©2020 Beck Institute for Cognitive Behavior Therapy. Reprinted from *beckinstitute.org* and used with permission. *Beck Institute (BI) is a nonprofit organization with the mission of improving lives worldwide through excellence in CBT. BI offers training in Cognitive Behavior Therapy and Recovery-Oriented Cognitive Therapy to health and mental health professionals around the world.*

Keeping to our core values during this season of change and stress will give our lives the meaning and purpose necessary, not simply to survive, but to flourish. The quote attributed to Socrates, "The unexamined life is not worth living," takes on a new meaning during a global crisis. Reflecting on "who" we are and "where" we ultimately want to go is an important, next step in the process.

CHAPTER 2

SELF-EMOTIONAL ASSESSMENT

To understand our personal reactions to the pandemic, it is important to review and assess our emotional, mental, and behavioral functioning prior to the crisis. Consider how effective your skills were for coping with conflict, managing moods, maintaining resiliency, and solving problems. Even if your pre-crisis skills and functioning were relatively positive and effective, you may still need to actively strengthen your adjustment and coping skills to handle the catastrophic level of pressures and living conditions that accompany the pandemic and its aftermath.

If you are aware of areas of your life that may not have been pleasant and effective pre-crisis, you may need to seek help with resources and support that can assist you in learning how to grow through the many problems of a major social and health crisis. You can also monitor your functioning as you deal with the pandemic, and after the crisis has passed.

There are tools that can measure mental, emotional, and behavioral functioning. Some self-administered tools are available for personal assessment. You may have some questions as you consider the results of your assessments. Some of the telephonic resources have toll free lines that offer brief support and consultation with callers. If you are enrolled in a health plan or employee assistance plan, there may be a telehealth service that you could consult for medical or psychological information and consultation as well.

The following links for self-assessment are available to you now:

Stress
CIGNA Stress Quiz and Plan for Action
https://www.cigna.com/takecontrol/tc/stress/

Anxiety
Anxiety test
A Snapshot report free, but a charge is made for a Full Report
https://www.psychologytoday.com/us/tests/health/anxiety-test

Depression
An 18 Question, Automated Quiz on Depression
https://psychcentral.com/cgi-bin/depression-quiz.cgi

Also, a 20-minute depression test, which determines whether you have or are at risk for developing depression, and whether your mindset makes you more prone to depression. You receive a snapshot report free, but a charge is made for a full report. www.psychologytoday.com/us/tests/health/depression-test

Family For Depression Awareness: Depression Test
http://familyaware.org/Moodtest/disclaimer.php

UCLA medical school posts a range of self-assessment instruments, including those for depression, anxiety, and stress.
Self-Assessments - Behavior Wellness Center - Los Angeles, CA

Resilience
Resilience Assessment tool - Innovative Leadership Institute https://www.innovativeleadershipinstitute.com/resilience-assessment-tool.html

Migraine headaches, heart attacks, strokes, high blood pressure, and respiratory issues all surge during a time of crisis. Assessing your "emotional state" is an important tool in minimizing the potential, negative health impact. Regardless, though, of the results of your "self-emotional assessment," an important, next step for all of us is in making a self-medical assessment.

CHAPTER 3

SELF-MEDICAL ASSESSMENT

Medical Testing - Positive or Negative for COVID-19 Infection

Several professional medical testing programs are being developed during the writing of this book. Efforts are being made to produce equipment and processes that can quickly determine whether you are positive or negative for the COVID-19 infection. The tests in development are designed to determine whether you had the virus and may now have antibodies and possibly be immune. The progress and products will be available to you on the CDC website. Production of tests that provide rapid results are expected.

Self-assessment also includes determination of whether or not we may be infected with the COVID-19 virus, based on symptoms and situations. There are several options for this self-screening. At the time of publication, some of the self-tests are listed here.

The **Coronavirus Self-Checker** is the Center for Disease Control's bot which can assess the symptoms and risk factors for people worried about infection, provide information, and suggest a next course of action such as contacting a medical provider or, for those who do not need in-person medical care, managing the illness safely at home. The bot doesn't make a diagnosis or offer treatment plans, but it is meant to act as a guide to help people discern if they should seek certain medical care." Testing for COVID-19, CDC.gov website

Amazon's Alexa voice assistant can help you diagnose COVID-19.

Queries such as "Alexa, what do I do if I think I have coronavirus?" or "Alexa, what do I do if I think I have COVID-19?" will prompt the voice assistant to ask about your symptoms, travel history, and possible exposure to the virus. It will then offer advice based on Centers for Disease Control and Prevention information.

Amazon's Alexa voice assistant can now help you diagnose COVID-19

Apple's COVID-19 website and **COVID-19 app** are resources to help people stay informed and take the proper steps to protect their health during the spread of COVID-19. It is based on the latest CDC guidance. It is available on the Apple App Store. They were created in partnership with the CDC, the White House Coronavirus Task Force, and FEMA, to make it easy for people across the country to get trusted information and guidance. The app and website allow users to answer a series of questions around risk factors, recent exposure, and symptoms for themselves or a loved one. In turn, they will receive CDC recommendations on next steps, including guidance on social distancing and self-isolating, how to closely monitor symptoms, whether or not a test is recommended at this time, and when to contact a medical provider. This new screening tool is designed to be a resource for individuals and does not replace instructions from healthcare providers or guidance from state and local health authorities. The app may be downloaded from the Apple App Store, at no cost.

CHAPTER 4

EXPERIENCING PHYSICAL QUARANTINE & ISOLATION

Efforts to limit the spread of the virus include quarantine and isolation. **Quarantine** is separating well people who have been exposed to the virus from other persons, to determine if they become ill. **Isolation** is separating persons who have illness symptoms so that they can't infect others, including close family members. These actions may be self-determined or determined by government officials.

When humans are separated, even in efforts to protect the health of others in the population, the circumstances can be very challenging. This is especially true when large groups of the population are separated. Some of the issues related to the separation and isolation experiences are:

Information may be limited or wrong
There is information overload, often with distrust of quality
    Sources of truth and accuracy are suspect.
Much information creates confusion, uncertainty, and anxiety
    Personal supplies may be inadequate or not available
    Difficulty planning and preparing
        Nutrition is difficult to maintain
    Financial loss and fear of loss adds strong concerns
        There can be a real or perceived stigma about being "sick."
    Loss of routines reduces a sense of personal structure and consistency

Boredom fuels depressed moods
  Frustration with limits and unpleasant conditions, quickly builds

Fear of infection or infecting others (esp. vulnerable family members) drives anxiety, shame, and guilt feelings

Less empathy or loss of expressed empathy, because of fear and anxiety

Loss of social and physical contact with others leaves a sense of isolation from others and the world

These issues and reactions have strong effects on all of us. The global impact of COVID-19 on all personal needs, can be graphically illustrated with psychologist Abraham Maslow's 1943 published theory of a hierarchy of needs. These needs are represented as a pyramid with more basic needs at the bottom. Of the five proposed basic needs, the two at the bottom are **physiological** and **safety** needs. Above those are love/belonging (connection), esteem, and self-actualization. Given the demands and difficulty of meeting physiological needs (food, hygiene, rest, etc.) and staying safe in the chaotic health, social, spiritual and financial elements of a pandemic, it is not difficult to see that many of us experience serious difficulty in finding food or toilet paper and are not able or desirous to give much time to daily meeting esteem and self-actualization needs.

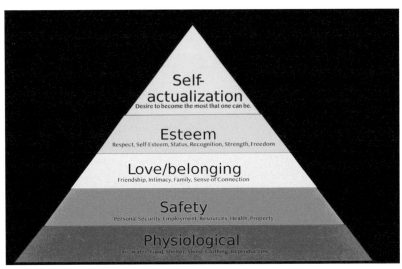

Maslow's Pyramid

When "normal" living conditions allow for functioning and meeting the needs of the first three levels, opportunities exist for attention to be given to higher levels of esteem and self-actualization.

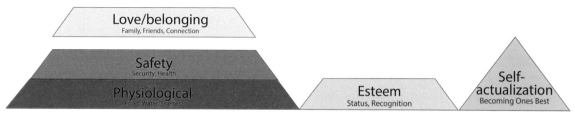

Distorted Maslow's Pyramid

Like building blocks that fall apart, we are overwhelmed by narrowly focused activities to meet critical and urgent needs such as finding food, medical and hygiene supplies, and in being careful of our medical safety, and the avoidance of infection or infecting others. In what feels like a crucible, opportunities and time do not allow for attention to more than basic needs. As the book cover displays, the virus has attacked and damaged the pyramid.

Nonetheless, it is possible to meet the love/belonging/connection needs through small group contacts, telephone calls, Skype, Facetime, Zoom, message texts, and email. Dr. Ellen Iverson, the Director of the Beck Institute's Recovery-Oriented Cognitive Therapy Training Program, writes about the need for connection:

"Connection is a basic human need (Baumeister & Leary, 1995) and the foundational component of Recovery-Oriented Cognitive Therapy (CT-R). Connection can involve having a sense of unity with another person or group of people, feeling like you belong or are a part of something bigger than yourself, and taking opportunities to share your values and talents with others (Beck et al, in press). The impact is significant: social disconnection correlates with poorer physical health—including shorter life expectancy (Green et al, 2018); withdrawal and isolation have been linked to increased rates of rehospitalization and longer inpatient psychiatric hospital stays for individuals with serious mental health conditions, such as schizophrenia (Patel et al, 2015); and social exclusion is connected to defeatist beliefs (e.g. "What's the point of trying, I will just fail anyway;" "Failing part way is the same as failing all the way;" Reddy, et al, 2017). How do we help facilitate connection when the prescription for the country is separation?" Ellen Iverson, Psy.D.,

Connection, Belonging, and Purpose in the World of Social Distancing, ©2020 Beck Institute for Cognitive Behavior Therapy. Reprinted from *beckinstitute.org* and used with permission.

Beck Institute is a nonprofit organization in Philadelphia that offers national and international training in Cognitive Behavior Therapy.

The difficulties meeting physiological, safety and belonging/connection needs are real and serious. Dr. Iverson is right—it is not easy to facilitate connection when our entire country is in separation. Often, in addition to unpleasant 'issues' of separation (as noted above), symptoms of psychological distress may appear when we are disconnected by quarantine, isolation, and voluntary confinement:

Mood disturbances—sadness or depression
Anxiety
Fear
Hopelessness
Post-traumatic stress symptoms
Irritability
Reduced ability to focus
Mental confusion
Emotional and physical fatigue
Sleep disturbance

The behavioral healthcare system has never witnessed before such a global concentration of these symptoms of psychological distress. It may have been W.H. Auden who first penned the phrase, "The Age of Anxiety," his Pulitzer Prize winning poem of 1948, which deals with our quest to find identity and meaning in an increasingly changing world. The four-character dramatic poem is set in a New York City bar during World War II. Today, our world has been turned upside down, and we need to examine our anxieties and fears if we are to successfully manage our lives in this new, "Age of Anxiety."

CHAPTER 5

ANXIETY AND FEAR

Our responses to COVID-19 include anxiety and fear. Those threats that are not clearly known or are possibly dangerous, trigger anxiety and personal responses to the stress of those thoughts and feelings. There are many things (stressors) in the pandemic that are unknown to us and can produce uncomfortable and sometimes debilitating symptoms. Concerns like "Do I have the virus?" "Where is the virus going to spread?" and "Is it safe to go to the store?" can result in acute physiological reactions and other symptoms. They come from your mind's interpretation of the possible dangers that could arise.

Fear is experienced when we know and understand the real threat that produces stress responses. Learning that you tested positive for COViD-19 infection presents a known and specific threat, and your fear response(s) can be similar to anxiety responses. Examples of fear and anxiety responses are:

Irritability
Headaches
Muscle pain and tension
Sleep disturbances
Tightness felt throughout the body, especially in the head, neck, jaw, and face
Chest pain
Ringing or pulsing in ears
Excessive sweating

Shaking and trembling
Cold chills or hot flushes
Accelerated heart rate
Numbness or tingling
Depersonalization
Upset stomach or nausea
Shortness of breath
Feeling like you're going insane
Dizziness or feeling faint.

Fears, anxieties, and these reactions can take an emotional toll, especially if you're already living with some difficulty with anxiety. The feelings can be, or seem to be, life threatening. At this intensity, we sometimes feel detached and the sympathetic branch of the autonomic nervous system is turned on and takes control, preparing us unconsciously for a "fight or flight" action. It is our wiring, designed to protect us from perceived threats, whether they are clearly known to be, or possibly could be dangerous.

Fear and anxiety produce similar responses to certain dangers. But there are important differences between the two. These differences represent how we can respond to the different stressors and manage our reactions. Responding to "real" threats calls for actions that help us avoid or minimize the danger to us. Learning that a close coworker tested positive for the virus can produce an intense fear-reaction, but isolating yourself and taking actions to sanitize yourself and your environment are evidence of working a plan to manage the fear.

Obsessively worrying (anxiety) about the "what ifs" of life in a lockdown, or at work, can produce many emotional and mental reactions with varied symptoms. But your management efforts can utilize mental and behavioral activities that work to reduce the stress reactions and can change your perception and understanding of the stressors. These stressors are no longer controlling you. You are controlling them by "managing your stress."

CHAPTER 6

MANAGING STRESS

Rethinking our stress response is a basic and critical foundation for managing stress reactions in difficult times. A tool that can help you re-evaluate our view of stress is *Rethinking Stress,* a series of videos and a workbook, by SparqTools. It is a research-based, self-paced, simplified video program from Stanford University. http://sparqtools.org/rethinkingstress/

Stress can also be defined as "When the demands we experience challenge our ability…or perceived ability…to meet those demands." Richard Lazarus, PhD.

What we call *"stress"* is made up of:

Stressors – anything that knocks us out of balance. All those things that bother us, pressure us, scare us, worry us, etc. are called stressors. They include external circumstances, as well as our own perspective, expectation, or attitude.

Stress-responses – what our body does to try to establish balance. How we react to those stressors is called our stress-response. It is how we try to get back into balance, while and after being hit with stressors. How we react to those stressors is called our stress-response.

Our stress-response is highly sensitized to:
 What resources do we have to help us?
 Do we see the stress as a threat, or can we see an opportunity?
 What habits do we have when we automatically respond (brain circuits)?

Stress is an engineering term. Literally, it's the force placed on an object. Internal stress (or 'strain') is the strength of the object to resist the forces against it. Think of yourself as a train bridge, having the strength and resilience to handle the stress of the heavy train straining your foundation and structure, to withstand its force.

How many stress events do you ordinarily have per day? Social psychology researchers estimate we have **30** stress "opportunities" per day, which equals ¾ million in a lifetime! Some of these stress opportunities include:

Daily Frustrations
Uncertainties
Demands
Deadlines
Disappointments
Tensions
Conflicts

Living in the COVID-19 social, medical, and personal environment significantly increases the number and intensity of daily stress opportunities.

Our usual responses to stressors tend to become habitual. How we automatically respond to these daily challenges predicts our mood, health, relationships, motivation and productivity. Our stress habits, whether they be good or bad, may have to be questioned and re-learned under the effects of the global pandemic. We can notice our emotional responses, our internal dialogue (self-talk), our behaviors, and thought processes in order to transform our stress reactions and become more resilient.

For many persons, it seems the COVID-19 stressors constantly set off a cascade of physiological, mental, and behavioral reactions (stress responses). In normal times, 60-80% of primary doctor visits have a stress component. Currently, given the increased stressors of the COVID-19 virus living conditions, it is not difficult to understand a major increase in stress responses. We can consider our level of stress by mentally focusing on our reactions and assigning a "stress number" on a zero to ten scale.

0 = total absence of stress or tension
10 = Panic attack

Stress is cumulative, and even though we may not be near the panic attack level, continuous stress builds and increases to a painful and damaging state. We need to hit the reset button and reduce or stop the building stress. To do this, you can challenge your negative stress thoughts.

Practice stopping in order to challenge your perceptions that are distressing:

1. Stop
2. Take a deep breath
3. Dispute or challenge your perceptions and expectations.

There are self-calming techniques that assist your nervous system in self-regulating:

1. Breathe slowly and deeply
2. Relax your muscles
3. Take inventory of your resources for assistance
4. Stretch your muscles
5. Listen to your self-talk
6. Focus inward and be Mindful of the moment
7. Meditate using pleasant thoughts
8. Visualize a scene that brings peace or happiness
9. Engage in Deep Relaxation
10. Do vigorous exercise

Calming with Deep breathing:

We take short shallow breaths when we're stressed
But deep abdominal breaths help us relax
Slow, deep, diaphragm breathing helps
Exhaling engages a calming, (PNS) response
Train self to do on-demand self-calming
Cue words help; "relax" "let go" "release." These can be paired with progressive muscle relaxation.

Additional Self-Calming Techniques include:

Tense-Release muscle relaxation
Play, laugh, smile
Dispute negative self-talk
Mindfulness
Other-focused helping
Acting out Values
Prioritize/organize pressures
Take control of what you can and let go of what you can't control

Regardless of the pressures of this new, COVID-19 world we live in, we have the ability and resources to manage our stress. The old Beatles song, "Let it Be," may be a good starting point. If we don't manage our stress, more serious behavioral health issues will result. Depression is one of them.

CHAPTER 7

DEPRESSION

Even with efforts to manage stress and stress reactions, it is common to experience sadness and depressed moods in life under COVID-19. Living conditions are complicated, frustrating, limiting, confusing, emotionally painful, and socially stressful. The emotion of sadness can be experienced relative to our sense of helplessness, disappointment in difficulty or time to control the virus, loss of pleasant living space/conditions, social distancing, etc. An old English meaning of sad was weary or weighted. It was replaced in Middle English by senses or emotions as "sorrowful." Today, we feel sad or sorrowful when we experience loss and inability to correct or fix a desired situation. It is an emotional pain that arises from the loss of a range of things, from personal freedom and pleasant living conditions to the loss of a loved one. In a generic sense, we all have losses that can result in sadness, and to some extent, grieving, or the acute pain associated with the loss.

In specific, the death of COVID-19 patients brings sadness and grief to the remaining loved ones. These feelings, along with possible anger, anxiety, denial, and confusion are complicated and overlaid with the remaining person's reactions to the COVID-19 impact. Such is the case for over 60,000 deaths in the U.S.to date.Lockdown at home and the lockout of hospitals and other medical facilities amplify our emotions around not being able to support or say goodbye to a dying loved one, and not knowing if anyone will be present when death occurs. Even grieving the loss of the loved one must be done in the midst of multiple stressors and other losses. For those of you experiencing the trauma of life in COVID-19 and also the trauma of a loved one dying (with none of the usual family opportunities before or after death), it can help to contact the emotional helplines or a healthcare professional for support, coaching, counseling, and possible assessment of your condition.

Clinical depression (major depressive disorder) is not the same as sadness or grieving. It is a complex medical condition that includes emotional, physical, and cognitive symptoms. There are three risk factors for developing clinical depression:

Personal or family history of depression
     Major life changes, trauma, or stress
     Certain physical illnesses and medications

COVID-19 and its medical and social management bring to many persons, major life changes, trauma and stress. Not everyone in this risk category will develop clinical depression, but it is important to monitor your moods and mental condition, as you continue to deal with the trauma and stress of living conditions under the pandemic. The material below is provided by the National Institute of Mental Health's public material.

Depression Signs and Symptoms

If you have been experiencing some of the following signs and symptoms most of the day, nearly every day, for at least two weeks, you may be suffering from depression:

     Persistent sad, anxious, or "empty" mood
     Feelings of hopelessness, or pessimism
     Irritability
     Feelings of guilt, worthlessness, or helplessness
     Loss of interest or pleasure in hobbies and activities
     Decreased energy or fatigue
     Moving or talking more slowly
     Feeling restless or having trouble sitting still
     Difficulty concentrating, remembering, or making decisions
     Difficulty sleeping, early-morning awakening, or oversleeping
     Appetite and/or weight changes
     Thoughts of death or suicide, or suicide attempts
     Aches or pains, headaches, cramps, or digestive problems without a clear physical cause

Not everyone who is depressed experiences every symptom. Some people experience only a few symptoms while others may experience many. Several persistent symptoms in addition to low mood are required for a diagnosis of major depression, but people with only a few – but distressing – symptoms may benefit from treatment of their minor symptoms of depression. The severity and frequency of symptoms and how long they last will vary depending on the individual and his or her particular illness. Symptoms may also vary depending on the stage of the illness.

Risk Factors

Depression is one of the most common mental disorders in the U.S. Current research suggests that depression is caused by a combination of genetic, biological, environmental, and psychological factors.

Depression can happen at any age, but often begins in adulthood. Depression is now recognized as occurring in children and adolescents, although it sometimes presents with more prominent irritability than low mood. Many chronic mood and anxiety disorders in adults begin as high levels of anxiety in children.

Depression, especially in midlife or older adults, can co-occur with other serious medical illnesses, such as diabetes, cancer, heart disease, and Parkinson's disease. These conditions are often worse when depression is present. Sometimes medications taken for these physical illnesses may cause side effects that contribute to depression. A doctor experienced in treating these complicated illnesses can help work out the best treatment strategy.

Risk factors include:

Personal or family history of depression
Major life changes, trauma, or stress
Certain physical illnesses and medications

Treatment and Therapies

Depression, even the most severe cases, can be treated. The earlier that treatment can begin, the more effective it is. Depression is usually treated with <u>medications</u>, <u>psychotherapy</u>, or a combination of the two.

Quick Tip: No two people are affected the same way by depression and there is no "one-size-fits-all" for treatment. It may take some trial and error to find the treatment that works best for you.

Psychotherapies

Several types of psychotherapy (also called "talk therapy" or, in a less specific form, counseling) can help people with depression. Examples of evidence-based approaches specific to the treatment of depression include cognitive-behavioral therapy (CBT), interpersonal therapy (IPT), and problem-solving therapy.

Beyond Treatment: Things You Can Do

Here are other tips that may help you or a loved one during treatment for depression:
Try to be active and exercise
Set realistic goals for yourself
Try to spend time with other people and confide in a trusted friend or relative
Try not to isolate yourself, and let others help you
Expect your mood to improve gradually, not immediately
Postpone important decisions, such as getting married or divorced, or changing jobs until you feel better.
Discuss decisions with others who know you well and have a more objective view of your situation.
Continue to educate yourself about depression.

If you're experiencing depression, get help, and get help now. Do not be afraid to reach out. Help is available. The resources and tools in this book are just a beginning. With help, you can manage your stress and depression. You're more resilient than you think!

CHAPTER 8

RESILIENCY

Resiliency is a quality that gives us the psychological strength to cope with trauma and stress. It allows us to bounce back after pressure and to continue functioning physically and emotionally. It is the personal element that supports our efforts to adjust our thinking and take necessary stress management actions. It prevents us from becoming emotionally drained and depleted. Resiliency allows us to remain calm in adversity, *like a kayaker who rights herself in the middle of the rapids.* We all have different levels of resiliency, but it is possible to learn how to build it and apply it. The following definitions of resilience, and characteristics of non-resilience are from Dr. Al Siebert's work in resilience.

Definitions:

Resilience, resilient, and resiliency refer to the ability to

- cope well with high levels of ongoing disruptive change;
- sustain good health and energy when under constant pressure;
- bounce back easily from setbacks;
- overcome adversities;
- change to a new way of working and living when an old way is no longer possible; and
- do all this without acting in dysfunctional or harmful ways.

Characteristics of Non-Resilient/ Poor Coping:
    Overreact to disruption (changes)

Don't contemplate the big picture
Dwell on negative feelings
Blame others – play the victim role
Don't trust – withdraw
Fearful – focus on worst case scenarios
External locus of control (helplessness)

From *The Resiliency Advantage*, Al Siebert, PhD, Berrett-Koehler Publishers, Inc. 2005, San Francisco, CA

How to build resiliency:

- Cherish social support and interaction. Good relationships with family and friends and others are vital.
- Treat problems as a learning process. Develop the habit of using challenges as opportunities to acquire or master skills and build achievement.
- Avoid making a drama out of a crisis. Stress and change are part of life.
- Celebrate your successes. Take time at the end of each day to review what went well and congratulate yourself.
- Develop realistic life goals for guidance and a sense of purpose.

Some additional suggestions to help you build your resilience

- Accept the unchangeable things as they are. Acceptance is a skill. The ability to accept the reality of a situation and understand what you are able to change is necessary for one's inner peace.
- Extend kindness to others. Practicing altruistic behavior can activate circuits in the brain that are key to one's well-being.
- Cultivate your relationships and connectivity. In a time of isolation, staying connected with supportive peers and family via video chat, text, email or a phone call may be the best antidote against the sadness and depression that can accompany isolation.
- Be decisive: Even in times of rapid change and enormous pressure, we can solve many of our problems by making smart and efficient decisions. Don't be afraid to act!

Resiliency is not a distinct talent given to a few. It is an acquired skill and can be learned. We need not be trapped in behavioral patterns of "poor coping" and "stress avoidance," which only generate more stress. Each of us carries within us the ability to adjust to change and meet new challenges. Some of us have more resilience than others, but we can all learn, develop, improve and practice our resiliency.

CHAPTER 9

MINDFULNESS

Mindfulness is our basic human ability to pay attention on purpose, in the present moment, and in a non-judgmental way. It is when we self-regulate our attention with openness. It is the ability to be fully present, aware of where we are and what we are doing, without overreacting or being overwhelmed with what is happening outside or around us. Our mind processes and constantly computes information about external circumstances and internal feelings. It is possible to control our awareness and focus it on the moment, being mindful without judgement. The goal of mindfulness is to wake up to the inner workings of our mental, emotional, and physical processes, and in being kind and forgiving of ourselves.

Living in the pandemic, we experience strange and difficult situations, fearful thoughts, and intense feelings. We are mostly reacting on autopilot. Using the technique or process of mindfulness allows us to occasionally decide to take time out and consider our external and internal states objectively, without self-criticism or overreacting. Doing this sends a message that we are not powerless. We may not be able to change the stress of external circumstances, but we have the power and control to change our perceptions and therefore reduce some of the internal stress reactions. Mindfulness and related interventions have shown to be effective with depression, anxiety and chronic pain. Cortisol is the "fight or flight" hormone that is triggered when we sense danger or experience stress. Some studies show that mindfulness can result in reduction of cortisol and our internal reactions: https://news.harvard.edu/gazette/story/2018/04/harvard-researchers-study-how-mindfulness-may-change-the-brain-in-depressed-patients/

In simple terms, we can decide to decide what to give attention to. Henry Ford said it many years ago, ""If you think you can or you can't, you're probably right."

The Mindfulness Research Data below can help you get through this stressful time:

In 2013, researchers at UC Davis discovered a very powerful connection between mindfulness and cortisol, with remarkable results seen within only a few short weeks. Cortisol, a major age-accelerating hormone, is the one chemical where less is better. Luckily, scientists have found a very powerful solution.

https://eocinstitute.org/meditation/how-meditation-reduces-your-ocd/

Mindfulness-Based Interventions for People Diagnosed with a Current Episode of an Anxiety or Depressive Disorder: Mindfulness-based stress reduction (MBSR) is a clinically standardized meditation that has shown consistent efficacy for many mental and physical disorders.

https://journals.plos.org/plosone/article?id=10.1371/journal.pone.0096110

Studies have shown benefits against an array of conditions both physical and mental areas — including depression, chronic pain, and anxiety — in which well-designed, well-run studies have shown benefits for patients engaging in a mindfulness meditation program, with effects similar to other existing treatments.

https://news.harvard.edu/gazette/story/2018/04/harvard-researchers-study-how-mindfulness-may-change-the-brain-in-depressed-patients/

You are not powerless. The tips in these websites can help you cope with the stressful times of the pandemic.

Here are some Techniques of Mindfulness:

- Body sensations: For five to ten minutes in the morning and/or evening, sit quietly and simply observe the physical sensations in your body. Label them as you notice them e.g., "Now squeezing," "Twisting," "Throbbing," or "Pulsating discomfort."
- Set your wristwatch or cell phone so that an alarm goes off every two to three hours to remind you to be mindful of the physical sensation in that moment.
- Emotions: Whenever an upsetting event arises during the day, pause and pay attention to what you're feeling physically. In contrast, whenever a happy event arises during the day, pause and pay attention to what you're feeling in your body.
- Sensory: Going barefoot opens up a world of sensory stimulation. It also comes with some really major awareness challenges. Be aware of various physical sensations and balance.
- Regulate your emotions, deciding for fun, laughter, and social contacts.
- Separate negative perceptions as real or imagined—see things as they really are.
- Attend to positive perceptions
- Identify your negative stress language under pressure;
  - "I'm stressed out."
  - "This is too much for me."
  - "I hate this situation. I can't take it."
  - "Why does this happen to me?"
- Practice positive stress language:
  - "It's not as bad as I am feeling."
  - "I can decide to do this."
  - "I can relax and control my feelings."

The above tips, techniques and websites can help you practice a "mindfulness" that can assist you in the most stressful of times. Mindfulness is what makes us fully human, fully alive. If it is true that in some sense the past, the present, and the future are one, then we are to live fully in the moment. It is the "now" that we have been given. Cherish it.

If you need and desire further help, the remaining chapters will provide you with a vast assortment of resources and services that are available to help you live a healthy, productive and meaningful life. Take this moment—"now"—to look through them and see if any of the offerings might be suitable for you or someone whom you love.

CHAPTER 10

PROFESSIONAL COUNSELING

When you need counseling or therapy, or a professional assessment of your mental and emotional condition, you may contact behavioral health professionals who are contracted with your health or EAP plan. The contact number is often printed on your insurance/health plan ID or eligibility card. Where a mental health or EAP number is not specified, you may call the number listed for medical services. Many of these plans are provided through your employer. If you do not have a health benefit program, or if you want to directly select a mental health provider, there are several organizations that provide networks of professionals that provide telehealth services. It is important to note that there are published fees for these services. The provider selected may not be contracted with the network provided by your health plan, making insurance reimbursement not usually available. Given the increased approvals for telehealth services and various financial assistance programs, it is important to verify these issues if you choose to have the professional services reimbursed.

Following is a partial list of behavioral health networks that make telehealth counseling available.

Disclosure: The providers are independent professionals. This book is limited to providing information only and does not assume responsibility or liability for services provided. Links exist to other websites and you are responsible to evaluate the content, services, and usefulness of connected or related sites.

Telehealth Groups:

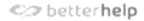

WellVia Behavioral Health solutions
- Psychiatrists and licensed counselors
- Secure and private online video and phone sessions
- Counseling, medication management and assessments
- Wellness services
- Coaching

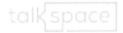

BetterHelp
- Over 4900 therapists, PhD, PsyD, LMFT, LCSW, LPC, LMSW
- Text messages, live chat, phone, video conference, app
- HIPAA compliant, secure, and anonymous

---

talk space

Talkspace
- Text, video and audio messaging
- Separate platform for teens and also couples
- 5,000 licensed, credentialed providers

ReGain-
- Focused exclusively on relationship counseling
- Two users/couples can share a joint account
- Therapists are all licensed professionals

 Faithful Counseling

Faithful Counseling
- Licensed therapists who are practicing Christians
- Phone, video, live chat, messaging
- Counseling from a biblical perspective

Pride Counseling
- Any gender, orientation, or identity in the LGBTQ community
- Therapists specialized in LGBTQ issues
- Anonymous and secure
- Phone, video, messaging, smartphone app

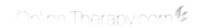

Online-Therapy.com

- Focused on Cognitive Behavioral Therapy (CBT)
- Self-help course with workbooks, activity plans, videos, and various tools
- Access to certified therapists via live chat, messaging

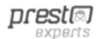

Presto Experts

- Pay by the minute; no subscription plan
- 20 therapists listed for "Anxiety and Stress"
- Patient chooses expert based on profiles

Wellnite

- Monthly visits by video or phone, and text support
- Medical doctors offering medications or CBT
- Treatment plan mapped out during initial visit with MD
- Monthly subscription includes cost of one prescription a month

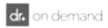

Doctor On Demand

- Psychiatry visits
- Therapy visits
- Visits are 15 minutes; can extend for additional fee
- Platform integrates to health plans

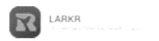

Larkr

- Text messaging and video; App-based
- Self-guided meditations, journaling, and mental health suggestions
- Therapy only; no prescriptions

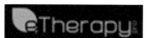

eTherapyPro

- Licensed therapists; nopsychiatrists; no prescribing
- App with voice, message, and video
- Patient is matched with a therapist

---

joyable

Joyable
- Coaches, not therapists
- Primarily designed for businesses and teams
- App-based coaching and therapy using CBT with online activities to reach goals

---

AmWell
- Licensed therapist visits
- Psychiatrist visits
- Web or app-based, with streaming video
- Psychiatrists will prescribe medications if appropriate

MDLIVE
- Medical doctor visits for a variety of physical conditions plus anxiety disorders
- For psychiatry appointments
- Phone or video
- Choose your doctor from the network directory

With telehealth, mental health workers provide their services through a telephone, internet video service, streaming media, video conferencing, or wireless communication. This online therapy is particularly useful for patients that live in remote rural locations that are far from institutions that provide mental health services. Currently, the national COVID-19 social and travel restrictions require telehealth services. Mental health providers that work in telehealth can only provide services to patients currently located in the state in which the provider is licensed, but some restrictions may be lifted during the COVID-19 pandemic.

TAKING CARE OF SELF AND OTHERS

FINANCIAL RESOURCE INFORMATION

Government programs are being developed and implemented to provide financial assistance:

2-1-1: Provides free and confidential information and referral. Call 2-1-1 for help with food, housing, employment, health care, counseling and more. http://www.211search.org/

Needy Meds: Provides help with the cost of medicine.
https://www.needymeds.org/

Modest Needs Foundation: Provides short-term financial assistance to individuals and families in temporary crisis.
https://www.modestneeds.org/for-applicants/apply-for-help.asp

CERF+ plays a unique role in providing emergency resources to the arts community. Tel: (802) 229-2306 https://cerfplus.org/

The Disaster Unemployment Assistance (DUA): Provides unemployment benefits to individuals who have become unemployed as a direct result of a Presidentially declared major disaster. 1-877-872-5627.

https://www.benefits.gov/benefit/597

Salvation Army: Provides financial assistance programs and resources.
https://www.salvationarmyusa.org/usn/covid19/

Energy bill assistance programs: Offered by utility companies.
https://www.needhelppayingbills.com/html/energy_assistance.html

Jewish interest free loan association:

https://www.needhelppayingbills.com/html/jewish_association_interest_fr.html

TELEPHONIC CRISIS and SUPPORT RESOURCES

When you need immediate support information or have a crisis, toll free telephone and text lines are available. If you or someone with you is in imminent danger with a life-threatening medical condition or possible suicide, you should call 911 directly.

Crisis Text Line:
Text "HELLO" to 741741

The Crisis Text hotline is available 24 hours a day, seven days a week throughout the U.S. The Crisis Text Line serves anyone, in any type of crisis, connecting them with a crisis counselor who can provide support and information.

Disaster Distress Helpline – SAMHSA:
Call 1-800-985-5990 24/7 via SMS, from the 50 states. Text **"TalkWithUs"** for English or "Hablanos" for Spanish to 66746. **Spanish-speakers from Puerto Rico can text "Hablanos" to 1-787-339-2663.**

Red Cross: If you have experienced a disaster and need extra support due to the new fears and stresses you may be feeling during this time, call the free, confidential SAMHSA Disaster Distress Helpline at 800-985-5990 or text TalkWithUs to 66746 to connect with a trained crisis counselor.

Home Numbers for State and Local Health Departments:
Health departments across the United States that travelers can use to connect with the health department in their destination state or the state they are in 1-800-CDC-INFO (800-232-4636) or TTY 888-232-6348.

Coronavirus Disease 2019 Questions:
In English or Spanish Mon. – Fri. 8 AM - 8 PM ET 800-CDC-INFO 800-232-4636

FEMA Disaster Assistance Helpline: Call 7 AM - 10 PM. ET, 7 days a week: 1-800-621-3362 (also for 711 & VRS) TTY 1-800-462-7585

FAMILY VIOLENCE:
Family Violence Prevention Center 1-800-313-1310

National Sexual Assault Hotline: 1-800-656-HOPE (4673)

National Domestic Violence Hotline: 1-800-799-SAFE, Spanish 1-800-942-6908

The Disaster Distress Helpline: Provides immediate crisis counseling for people who are experiencing emotional distress related to any natural or human-caused disaster. The helpline is free, multilingual (30 languages), confidential, and available 24 hours a day, seven days a week.

211: Connects millions of people to help every year. To get expert, caring help, simply call 211. http://www.211.org/

National Domestic Violence Hotline: Available 24hours and seven days a week, confidential, free of cost, Call 1-800-799-SAFE (7233) https://www.thehotline.org/help

LONELINESS HELPLINES:
Institute on Aging's Friendship Line is a 24-hour toll-free accredited crisis line 800-971-0016 https://www.ioaging.org/services/all-inclusive-health-care/friendship-line

Samaritans: sad, lonely, hopeless, or suicidal? The **Helpline** is available 24 hours a day, 7 days a week. Services are free, confidential, and anonymous.
HELPLINE: (877) 870-4673 https://samaritanshope.org/our-services/247-crisis-services/

CrisisTextLine: Helps to deal with **isolation and loneliness**: Text HOME to 741741 to connect with a Crisis Counselor https://www.crisistextline.org/topics/loneliness/

DOMESTIC ABUSE RESOURCES:
National Domestic Violence Hotline:
24/7 availability, confidential and free of cost. Provides life-saving tools and immediate support to enable victims to find safety and live lives free of abuse. 1-800-799-SAFE (7233). https://www.thehotline.org/

VictimConnect Resource Center : Where crime victims can learn about their rights and options confidentially and compassionately.855-484-2846.
https://victimconnect.org/get-help/talk-to-someone/

National Domestic Violence Hotline: Advocates are available for victims and anyone calling on their behalf to provide crisis intervention and safety. Call: 1-800-799-SAFE (7233) or TTY 1-800-787-3224. planning,https://www.bwjp.org/resource-center/resource-results/the-national-domestic-violence-hotline.html

Family and Youth Service Bureau: Immediate link to lifesaving help for victims. Hotline can be accessed via the nationwide number TTY, 1–800–787–3224 or (206)518-9361. https://www.acf.hhs.gov/fysb/programs/family-violence-prevention-services/programs/ndvh
ChildhelpLine: The Childhelp National Child Abuse Hotline is dedicated to the prevention of child abuse. All calls are confidential. Call 1-800-4-A-CHILD (1-800-422-4453) for help. https://www.childhelp.org/

CHAPTER 12

DIGITAL INFORMATION

Many organizations offer tips and mental health information on line and allow printing of fact sheets. These can be very convenient and helpful to review in the home setting, and to share with others.

NIMH - brochures and fact sheets on mental health disorders and related topics for patients and their families, health professionals, and the public. Printed materials can be ordered free of charge. Brochures and fact sheets are also offered in digital formats and are available in **English and Spanish**. https://www.nimh.nih.gov/health/publications/index.shtml

NIMH: Here are 5 steps you can take to **#BeThe1** To help someone in severe emotional pain and possibly suicidal:
https://www.nimh.nih.gov/health/publications/5-action-steps-for-helping-someone-in-emotional-pain/index.shtml

COVID-19 Lockdown Guide: How to Manage Anxiety and Isolation During Quarantine
https://adaa.org/learn-from-us/from-the-experts/blog-posts/consumer/covid-19-lockdown-guide-how-manage-anxiety-and

Managing Your Media-driven Anxiety:
https://www.anxiety.org/8-ways-to-manage-anxiety-and-stress-about-coronavirus

CDC: The nation's health protection agency, working 24/7 to protect America from health and safety threats, both foreign and domestic. CDC increases the health security of our nation. https://www.cdc.gov/coronavirus/2019-nCoV/index.html

Coping with COVID-19 News:
https://www.apa.org/helpcenter/pandemics

COVID-19 Legal Update: The Latest on the Novel Coronavirus' Impact on Businesses and Public Agencies
https://www.bbklaw.com/news-events/insights/2020/legal-alerts/03/covid-19-legal-updates

COVID-19 General Resources: American Psychological Association
https://www.apa.org/practice/programs/dmhi/research-information/pandemics

NASP public with information, guidelines, and resources to help support the learning and well-being of students, their families and others in the school community during the COVID-19 crisis. COVID-19 Resource Center

Disaster Communication and Resources:
https://www.apa.org/practice/programs/dmhi/research-information/disaster-communication

American Red Cross: Extensive information on planning and preparing. https://www.redcross.org/get-help/how-to-prepare-for-emergencies.html

Ad Council: in partnership with the federal government, public health partners, board member companies, major media networks and digital platforms http://coronavirus.adcouncilkit.org/

COVID-19 AND SOCIAL ISOLATION RESOURCES:
https://www.endsocialisolation.org/covid19

Monthly Webinars - Anxiety and Depression Association of America:
Free monthly webinars address some of the most frequently asked questions about psychological and pharmacological treatment of anxiety disorders, depression, and related disorders for adults as well as children. Experts offer tips and other information you need to know.
https://adaa.org/learn-from-us/from-the-experts/webinars

CHAPTER 13

EMOTIONAL HELP LINES

The National Network of Depression Centers (NNDC)
By calling 1-800-273-TALK (8255), you'll be connected with a skilled, trained counselor at a *crisis center* in your area, anytime 24/7.
https://nndc.org/resource-links/

MentalHelp.net provides online mental health and wellness education. Call the *Helpline* Toll-FREE 1-8663070990
https://www.mentalhelp.net/depression/unipolar-varieties/

American Psychological Association: *Crisis Hotlines Specialists* are available for confidential telephone counseling. National Suicide Prevention Lifeline (800) 273-8255 https://www.apa.org/helpcenter/crisis

American Psychological Association: *Crisis Text Line*
Text HELLO to 741741. Warm Line, free phone service offering mental health support,not intended for emergency situations. https://www.nami.org/NAMI/media/NAMI-Media/BlogImageArchive/2020/NAMI-National-HelpLine-WarmLine-Directory-3-11-20.pdf

Help Guide: *Mental health & wellness*
https://www.helpguide.org/home-pages/depression.htm

DBSA : *Depression and Bipolar Support Alliance*: offers in-person and online support groups.

https://www.dbsalliance.org/support/chapters-and-support-groups/find-a-support-group/

MedicineNet is an online, healthcare media publishing company. An interactive website. https://www.medicinenet.com/depression/article.htm

Psychology Today is a broad information source.
https://www.psychologytoday.com/us/basics/depression

Peer Support groups:
Support Group Central
https://www.supportgroupscentral.com/

The Anonymous Support Network
https://www.supportiv.com

Warm Line: A free phone service offering mental health support, not intended for emergency situations. https://www.nami.org/NAMI/media/NAMedia/BlogImageArchive/2020/NAMI-National-HelpLine-WarmLine-Directory-3-11-20.pdf

Help Guide: *Mental health & wellness*
https://www.helpguide.org/home-pages/depression.htm

DBSA: *Depression and Bipolar Support Alliance*: offers in-person and online support groups. https://www.dbsalliance.org/support/chapters-and-support-groups/find-a-support-group/

MedicineNet: An online, healthcare media publishing company. An interactive website. https://www.medicinenet.com/depression/article.htm

Psychology Today: An information source. https://www.psychologytoday.com/us/basics/depression

Care for Your Mind: Provided by Families for Depression Awareness, a national nonprofit organization providing training, advocacy, and programs for family caregivers of people living with depression or bipolar disorder. http://careforyourmind.org/depression-treatment-series/

CHAPTER 14

ACTIVITIES

With the "down time" of pandemic social effects, it is possible to take advantage of activities that are enjoyable and help focus yourself and others outward. Some suggestions are:

Explore: It's growing library consists of more than 250 original films and 30,000 photographs from around the world. https://explore.org/livecams

Calmsound: Nature sounds are recorded at the highest standards, allowing you to relax and enjoy the sounds of nature in all their glory.
https://www.calmsound.com/

Open Culture: Online courses from the world's top universities for free. http://www.openculture.com/freeonlinecourses

The Kennedy Center: Explore the video library of performing arts.
https://www.kennedy-center.org/digita lstage/digital-library/
ApplyFilter/?activeTab=MillenniumStage&sortColumn=PublishDate&sortDirection=Descending

Workout videos for every fitness level. Free.
https://www.fitnessblender.com/

Humanities Courses: Learn about the humanities and more.
https://www.edx.org/course/subject/humanities

LibriVox: Free public domain audiobooks.
https://librivox.org/

CHAPTER 15

RELIGIOUS HELPLINES

In times of personal crisis, our spiritual place and connection to God may be challenged or questioned. Contacting your religious organization may be possible through help or support lines. Priests, pastors, rabbis, and imans can be a source of understanding and spiritual assistance. If you don't have existing religious connections, several organizations offer 24-hour helplines.

CATHOLIC:

The Upper Room Crisis Hotline is a compassionate faith-based hotline with a Catholic Tradition. Call 1-888-808-8724 - 24 hrs a day – 7 days a week https://www.catholichotline.org/prayer-line

Priest Hotline: phone number is 888-808-8724 https://www.morrisherald-news.com/2015/05/14/religious-hotline-service-will-take-calls-from-all-customers/afxgzuz/

JEWISH

Jewish Helpline is a lifeline for those with nowhere to turn. Jewish Helpline can be reached on *0800 652 9249 www.jewishhelpline.co.uk*

The JQ Helpline: The free and confidential JQ Helpline provides customized support and inclusive resources over the phone, by email, and in person to those in need. Call 855.574.4577 https://jqinternational.org/about/

PROTESTANT:

Billy Graham Association 1-800-759-0700
Grace Help Line 24 Hour Christian service 1-800-982-8032
Need Encouragement: Call: 800-633-3446 https://needencouragement.com/

CHAPTER 16

WHEN LOSS, GRIEF AND PAIN BECOME PERSONAL

While working on *COVID-19: Resources for Coping with the Pandemic and Beyond*, I also have been grieving the death of my dear wife, Arlene, who passed away on December 11, 2019. She and I had been married sixty-one years, having been sweethearts since our university days in 1956.

While Arlene didn't die from the coronavirus that became a world-wide pandemic in March of 2020, like many others who have lost loved ones to Covid-19, I have been grieving her loss constantly. Loss and grief spares no one. They are central to our common humanity. And the pain that accompanies them can be excruciating. I share my personal story of loss in hopes of ameliorating some of that acute pain that accompanies loss and grief, and to encourage those brave caregivers who not only work on the front lines, but also those who work unnoticed, quietly caring for the sick and the dying and the recovering in the privacy of their homes.

Arlene's illness began over seven years ago. Her symptoms included severe memory loss, some Parkinson's activity, visual hallucinations, paranoid thoughts, fear, anxiety, and hostility. Along the way, she lost most of her vision from shingles concentrated in one eye and macular degeneration in the other eye.

Prior to the disease, Arlene had been an active and loving wife, mother and grandmother. She was a great cook and hostess, and a huge support to me as I traveled throughout the nation in my work. She was actively involved in church home groups, and helped develop a vibrant women's ministry at our local church in Pasadena, CA.

Initial indications of the disease were a series of Parkinson reactions, including severe muscle jerks and night terrors. This was followed by memory loss. She was soon evaluated, and early treatment was started with a brilliant research neurologist, Dr. Shankle. A spinal fluid assessment indicated extremely high and abnormal substances that damage the brain and impair the processing of information. It was then that the diagnosis of Lewy Body Dementia was confirmed, the same neurodegenerative disease that took the lives of musician Glen Campbell and the brilliant actor/comedian Robin Williams (Mr. Williams chose to end his life by suicide, prior to losing all of his faculties from this debilitating disease).

In Arlene's case, intravenous medications, oral medications, and a potent medication delivered in the form of a skin patch were all employed to "control" the disease, as there is no cure for it yet. All of this treatment was being done at home, and even though her symptoms improved somewhat, the medications targeted to boost her immune system had to be moved from the IV to a nasal infusion since the veins could no longer support the intravenous activity, resulting in a severe irritation from the adhesive of the skin patch, which subsequently required its termination. But, not unlike the Herculean efforts to find an antidote and cure for Covid-19, numerous friends and professionals came to our assistance to help us provide the best possible care and treatment we could for Arlene.

Two caring and supportive pharmacists who operate a small local pharmacy, took an unusual interest in Arlene's treatment and figured out a way to get the irritating, patch-based medication compounded into a dispenser that allowed direct placement on the skin with no irritation. That process is now being used for several other dementia patients!

Over the years, the pharmaceutical industry has taken a great deal of criticism for the high costs of medications. Much of this criticism is legitimate. There are opportunistic people and companies in every industry. But on the whole, we have the foundational elements for the best heath care in the world, and our pharmaceutical companies spend enormous sums in research and development to provide us with the needed drugs to cure disease and sustain life. While companies need to be held accountable for any malfeasance, and while specific, systemic changes need to be looked at carefully, we can be thankful that thousands of researchers, scientists, technicians and pharmacists are working tirelessly to provide palliative and curative drugs for Covid-19 and any of its permutations that might follow.

But even with the best pharmaceutical and medical support available to us, Arlene developed frightening visual hallucinations, reoccurring delusions that something or someone was harming or killing her, accompanied by rapid, uncontrolled hand and arm movements, and, eventually, times of acute aspiration due to the debilitation and malfunction of her throat muscles.

As my son, Dr. Brian Mayhugh, and I were working on this resource book, I couldn't help but reflect on two, distinct parallels of Arlene's final weeks of life to the final weeks for so many patients with COVID-19: In those closing weeks and days, Arlene was unable to eat and eventually her respiratory system shut down altogether. Simply put, she could no longer swallow and soon could no longer breathe. And so, it is true of COVID-19 patients. Literally, the breath of life is taken from them, and even when provided by a respirator, many no longer have the strength to fully intake and absorb the air provided to them. It is a heartless and cruel death. And therein is the other parallel to the diseases. There comes a time when all hope of recovery is lost. In Arlene's case, it came quietly early one morning, when she whispered to me, "I am going to die. I can't do anything. Please, let me die." Of course, because of the highly contagious nature of COVID-19, it is an especially heartless disease in forcing its victim to die in isolation and providing little if any closure for family and friends. At least Arlene and I could say a final goodbye.

I knew the "reality" of Arlene's disease when her primary physician told me that she might have twelve or so months to live. But even with that grim prognosis, by virtue of my faith, I prayed for a miracle…that God might heal her. Many of those prayers were at night, when Arlene would wake in a state of confusion and pronounced anxiety. Then miraculously, from my perspective, Arlene had fewer and less intense emotional disturbances and hallucinations. She was now able to sit with the family after dinner and watch television without the chaotic reactions she'd previously experienced. For that respite, I found myself saying, "Thanks be to God!" It was such a joy to see Arlene have some relief from her acute symptoms, and I and the family had forgotten how relaxing an hour or two of TV, even banal TV can be!

Sometimes in the midst of this devastating pandemic, we forget that thousands of people *are* recovering! If a 108 year-old-man in Albuquerque, New Mexico, can survive Covid-19, it would appear anything is possible! The challenge is this: we live in a disposable culture, and this novel disease we call Covid-19 preys on our elderly with a seemingly insatiable appetite. Our senior-citizen homes have been particularly vulnerable, with a substantial percentage of our Covid-19 deaths taking place there. Additionally, the African-American population has been disproportionately affected. In many ways, our nation is going through a period of profound, moral testing. Long after the Covid-19 virus abates and we anxiously await the arrival of its permutations, the great moral question of our time will remain: will we choose to care for the most vulnerable among us and fulfill those ancient words, that "whatever you did for one of the least of these my brothers and sisters of mine, you did for me." (Mathew 25:40 NIV)

We are never to give up hope, and never to stop putting that hope into practice by caring for the most weak and vulnerable among us. And while Arlene's respite from the ravages of Lewy Body Dementia was temporary in nature, it taught me never to give up hope.

It was during one of our regular scheduled visits with Dr. Shankle that he asked me if I would consider Arlene having another spinal assessment done, since she was already outliving the normal life expectancy for this supposed "final stage" of the disease. I was concerned that her physical and mental condition might make the spinal tap difficult, even dangerous, but, with his encouragement, I agreed to the procedure and arrangements were made with the hospital. As Arlene was being admitted to the pre-op area, an attentive physician arrived and literally took charge in prepping her, pushing her gurney down the hallway to the radiology department, helping her onto the table, and then taking her back to the discharge area when the procedure was completed. All the while, I was watching in wonderment and delight, along with the nurses, to see a senior physician serving a patient in such an attentive manner. (How many just such wonderful and caring physicians have we seen sacrificially working to end this Covid-19 pandemic!) Words of comfort soon came as this kind doctor told me that "everything went fine, and Arlene is going to be okay."

Several weeks later, I drove Arlene to Hoag Hospital (along with her trusty wheelchair) to see Dr. Shankle and obtain the spinal-fluid test results. When we entered his office, he was standing beside a large computer screen, staring intently at it and then back to us. His first words to me and Arlene were, "It's a miracle!" I was not accustomed to hearing the word "miracle" from seasoned medical personnel, and I had no idea why Dr. Shankle was saying that. The good doctor then swung the screen around and showed me the results from the spinal-fluid test done three years earlier versus the most recent test results. In simple terms, two types of "bad materials" (proteins) were identified in both tests. Both were extremely high and abnormal in the first test. One type remained extremely high and abnormal in the most recent test. The second type had dropped to a normal level. The doctor explained that this second type, when found in the spinal fluid, is expected to increase 10% each year until death. Arlene's test had dropped to normal, the basis for what Dr. Shankle termed "a miracle."

Arlene didn't leave the office that day completely healed. Many who have recovered from Covid-19 may not be completely healed. Many will continue to have respiratory and several other issues for years to come. Some experts predict that complete and permanent immunity may not be possible, but as Arlene and I left the good doctor's office that day, I sensed that something miraculous had transpired. This precious gift that we call life had been extended for our dear Arlene, allowing her to be with us for several more years. And during this extended time, she was given another gift, one that none of us saw coming—the gift of song.

Arlene began to spontaneously sing the old hymns and choruses of her youth. As is often the case in dementia patients, melodies and their accompanying words may be vividly recalled while little else is remembered. In Arlene's case, we were amazed because she was neither an energetic nor perfectly tuneful singer in the past, only reluctantly and quietly joining in on the singing during a Sunday morning church service. Now she was remembering and singing the verses and choruses of her favorite songs in near perfect pitch and with deep emotion. While otherwise being nearly incommunicado, her greatest joy came from singing her "favorites" throughout the day. One of those favorites was a simple chorus with a simple story to tell:

Did anybody tell you I love you today?
Put me on your list, let me be the first, I love you today!
God loves you and I love you and that's how it should be!

Before long, some of the caregivers started singing this song and several others that they had learned from hearing Arlene sing them over and over. What a tonic music can bring to an aching heart! Since ancient times, its soothing power has served as an antidote for emotional and physical pain. When King Saul found himself overwhelmed by depression, it was the young shepherd boy David—the songster and harp player—whom Saul called to court to comfort him in his darkest moods and alleviate his suffering.

So, do yourself this favor: surround yourself and those you care for with music. It doesn't matter what kind of music it is—whether it's Mozart or Miles Davis, Beyoncé or Bach, a polka band or the Women's Balkan Chorus, let music do its mysterious magic and be a healing agent in the midst of your loss, grief and pain. In Arlene's case, a wonderful peace would fill the room when she and her friends and caregivers would sing together. How those old hymns would lift Arlene's spirit! Whoever wrote that anonymous little chorus, "Did Anybody Tell You I Love You Today?" had no idea of the enormous comfort his or her music would provide Arlene from the discomfort of this bewildering, mind-bending disease.

Toward the end, while I was giving Arlene her morning infusion treatment, she began humming a familiar tune to another old gospel hymn of disputed authorship, "Farther Along," made even more famous by Elvis Pressley, Johnny Cash and the Willie Nelson versions. The song questions the prosperity of those who do evil, and the suffering of those who do good:

Farther along, we'll know all about it,
Farther along, we'll understand why;
Cheer up my brother, live in the sunshine,
We'll understand it all by and by.

A portion of the second verse seems particularly apt to our times:

> *Death has come and taken our loved ones,*
> *It leaves our home so lonely and drear….*

Whatever solace there may be in the sentiment of one of Arlene's "favorites," many people are tired of the tropes and clichés and pundits who promise us little hope while pointing an accusing finger at others. Many of us have grown weary and travelled long enough with the uncertainty and anxiety that accompany COVID-19, and by the loss, grief and pain we've experienced with the passing of family and friends. But by working together for the common good and by staying true to our core values, there might well be some important things we *will* understand better in the by and by: the cause, not only of Arlene's deadly disease and of COVID-19, but the cause of many other debilitating and deadly diseases; we *will* understand better the palliative *and* curative procedures, technologies, and medicines that will bring dignity to death and real hope for complete healing. And perhaps, just perhaps, we will understand the most important thing of all—that when one person suffers, we all suffer; and then, we will joyfully work together to help "the least of these" among us.

If we can understand these things and work toward these solutions, we will not have passed through this trying time in vain.

AFTERWORD

The scourge of COVID-19 is far from over. The virus is mercurial and opportunistic in nature, and it may yet again flourish in different areas and at various seasons.

Additionally, persons coming out of quarantine and isolation, both medically mandated and self-imposed, will have to cope with continuing frustrations, anxieties, and fears that have arisen around the social and medical mitigation of the pandemic. It's stressful to be separated from others, particularly those we love, and, particularly if a healthcare provider thinks you may have been exposed to COVID-19 and you show no symptoms. Other stresses are associated with the financial impact on employers and employees, and on our social and spiritual lives.

Everyone feels differently after quarantine with many mixed emotions, but some of the emotional reactions to coming out of quarantine *and* isolation may include:

- A deep sense of relief and gratitude.
- Fear and worry about your own health and the health of your loved ones.
- Stress from the experience of continuing to monitor yourself, or being monitored by others, for signs and symptoms of COVID-19.
- Sadness, anger, or frustration because friends or loved ones have unfounded fears of contracting the disease from contact with you, even though you have been determined not to be contagious.
- Guilt about not being able to perform normal work or parenting duties during quarantine.

- Emotional and mental health changes, including acute mood swings.
- Additionally, children may have a strong emotional reaction and be upset when they, or someone they know, has been released from quarantine or isolation.

With helpful recommendations to address a sense of grief that accompanies our emotional reactions to COVID-19 and its aftermath, Dr. Seth Gillihan posted an article on WebMD's blog on March 27, 2020, entitled: *Grieving the Loss of Life as We Knew It.* Dr. Gillihan is a licensed psychologist, author, and host of the weekly *Think Act Be* podcast. The article can be found at: https://blogs.webmd.com/mental-health/20200327/grieving-the-loss-of-life-as-we-knew-it. WebMD Blog © 2020 WebMD, LLC. All rights reserved.

It is clear that even after the worst of the pandemic is over, life will be something "new," though hardly "normal." The tension between "regulations" and "personal liberties" will be ongoing. Conflicts in our "basic values" will polarize and affect everyone from the President and Congress, to state, county, and city officials. The dynamic of this tension will be played out daily in the media and on our streets.

Elements of our ongoing, daily lives will continue to have stressors related to these personal restrictions, with their reduced opportunities for social involvement. Can you imagine living in a world where a handshake is obsolete? Yet, our response to these new challenges in a post-pandemic world will make all the difference. Although it will be more difficult to achieve, Maslow's Pyramid of basic needs—physiological (physical)/safety/love/belonging(connecting)—will continue to be possible. These basic, human needs will not go away. They are what bind us.

Drawing upon all of our emotional, mental and spiritual resources, we can play a major role in determining what our new life patterns will be. And in spite of our "social distancing," there are some things we can continue to *hold* onto: to our values, to our faith, and to the love we show to one another.

ABOUT THE AUTHORS

Dr. Sam Mayhugh, is an executive psychologist who recently retired from IBH, a behavioral healthcare company he founded over 30 years ago. His professional life has also been spent in private practice, in hospitals and outpatient offices. He graduated from Olivet Nazarene University and Purdue University. His PhD is from Indiana State University. He attended post doctorate certificate programs at Harvard and Oxford University. He has authored five works, including *C.I.P. Counseling Interaction Profile* (Association for Productive Teaching, 1969), co-authored the text, *Managed Behavioral Health Care, an Industry Perspective,* with Sharon A. Shueman, Ph.D. and Warwick G. Troy, PhD, MPH, (Charles C. Thomas, Springfield, Illinois, 1994, *Harold's Story – A Journey of Uncommon Healing,* (Trilogy Christian Publishers, 2019), and the soon-to-be released, *The Odyssey of King David – God's Broken Vessel.*

Dr. Sam also spent 7 years as a psychologist and special contractor with the United States Department of Homeland Security, helping prepare the country for bad actors, i.e. shooters and terrorists. The country is now facing invisible threats that are more deadly, relative to proportions of persons affected. We were not prepared for the extent and intensity of the Covid-19 pandemic. This book provides resources and assistance to persons wanting to learn about options to cope with and promote well-being, during and after the COVID19 crisis.

Dr. Brian Mayhugh is a psychologist and healthcare executive with 30-years experience in employee assistance, managed care, and the behavioral health industry. He currently serves as the Chief Clinical Officer for IBH. He has served on the IBH executive team for the past 30 years. He has a doctorate in psychology from Fuller Theological Seminary. He co-authored *The Development and Maintenance of Provider Networks*, in *Managed Behavioral Health Care, An Industry Perspective*, with Samuel Mayhugh, PhD, Sharon A. Shueman, PhD and Warwick G. Troy, PhD, MPH. (Charles C. Thomas, Springfield, Illinois, 1994, His special expertise includes crisis intervention, health benefits, senior executive leadership, and corporate safety issues.

Printed in the United States
By Bookmasters